# A Stroke of Hope

Other books by John O'Melveny Woods

*Return to Treasure Island*

*Lost Tomb of Alexander*

*Jesse James Secret*

*The Crusaders*

*A Stroke of Hope*

Also Available with Co-Author Frank Kelso

*California Gold*

*Juan's Revenge*

# A Stroke of Hope

## Essential Steps to Survive *and* Recover from Strokes

John O'Melveny Woods

Published by Intellect Publishing



ASOH-7



Contact the Author at

JohnWoods7@hotmail.com

www.JohnWoodsAuthor.com

# Disclaimer

First of all, I am not a medical practitioner. And that is the good news. Since I am not medically trained, I am not controlled, restrained or governed as to what I can say or not say.

I am a researcher, and patient. The stories I share are from firsthand knowledge or research I have personally conducted and are strictly my personal opinions.

I invite you to conduct your own research and then make an informed decision as to how to proceed with health treatments for yourself or someone you love.

As an aside, I believe one can only make an informed decision once they have been exposed to ALL sides and facts of an issue. It is important to me to simply present the information I believe to be true.

What you do after that is up to you.

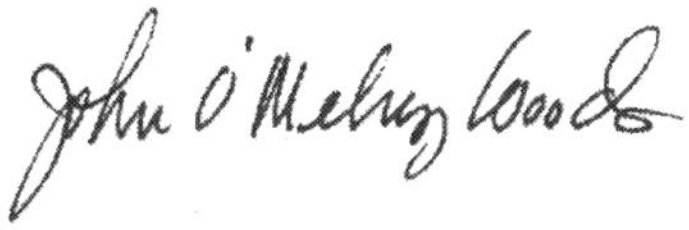

# A Stroke of Hope

## Essential Steps to Survive *and* Recover from Strokes

Stroke.

Most people don't give it a second thought. We hear about them all the time.

"Did you hear Larry had a stroke?"

"No, is he okay?"

In hushed tones they whisper: "He's in the hospital, paralyzed on one side and blind."

"Sorry to hear that."

Sorry to hear that. That's all it is to most of us. Hearing about it. Experiencing it firsthand is different. Much different. And then all the stories we've heard about strokes become real. Terrifyingly real.

What started out as a slight pain in my temples after a night of dinner and celebrating my wedding anniversary, escalated until it progressed into the most painful headache I had ever experienced.

It was a little after midnight. I had been tossing and turning for an hour. I screamed out as the pain continued to escalate, and then a horrible thought hit me: *Maybe I am dying.* I was 65, in pretty good health, and had no prior symptoms. But there I was, something going terribly wrong.

*I must get out of bed*, I thought. Standing up, I fell over in a dizzying spin. Plop, onto the floor I hit. *What is wrong with me?* I grasped the side of the bed, pulled myself up and fell back onto the mattress. *What? What?*

I called out for my wife. "Help! Judy, help!" She came rushing into the bedroom (she was sleeping in the other room due to a cold).

"Call an ambulance!" I cried out.

"What's wrong?" she asked.

"I don't know," I said. "I'm spinning. Dizzy. Something's wrong."

My wife bolted up the stairs to the house phone and dialed 911.

*Please don't let me die, God. Not yet. Don't let me die.*

It's funny how long-ago lost memories come back at the least expected times. I've always heard that when you are dying, your life 'flashes' before you. In my case, it played more like a movie

I was raised Catholic, altar boy, first communion, the works. But an incident with a priest who threw me out of a classroom by my ear in the 5th grade soured me on religion, an event from which I thought I would never recover. And yet, there I was in the bed, my head spinning like a sailor on a drunken binge, the worst headache of my life, Judy calling paramedics, and my first thought was *God, do not let me die*. Automatically reverting to my early Vatican beliefs. It didn't help that my mother was once a nun.

*God do not let me die.*

I heard Judy on the phone. She gave the address, followed by a long pause. Turns out we never had our location changed on the Internet phone we had in San Diego, and the 911 service routed her to San Diego. They gave her a different number. She called it. Thankfully, the San Diego dispatcher had already forwarded the address to Fairhope 911 and an ambulance was dispatched and on the way.

It took about fifteen LONG minutes for the emergency vehicle to arrive. Judy sat with me, holding my hand, which helped. I was floating in and out, spinning, and her touch tethered me to reality. I kept thinking, *Is this it? Am I going to die? Was I ready to die? Who is ready to die?*

*Maybe if they get me to the hospital in time, I will be alright.*

A knock on the door brought some hope. *Maybe if they get me to the hospital in time, I will be all right*. I heard voices and the clank of the metallic gurney coming toward the bedroom. Two young men appeared. They asked me what was wrong.

"I'm ... I'm dizzy."

"Can you stand up?"

"No."

"Okay, we'll help you onto the gurney."

They helped me sit up, which increased the pain in my head, and I squelched the urge to scream. They half dragged/carried me to the gurney and laid me down. The short litter ride to the ambulance through the house and onto the driveway was a blur. I didn't want to close my eyes, as if keeping them open would mean something. I didn't know what, but it was a hope to hold onto.

I was pushed through the rear door. The legs of the gurney clicked up and closed. As I observed the ceiling of the ambulance, one of the attendants took my temperature while the other fumbled for a package. He pulled out an IV while the other one then took my blood pressure. The first fellow dropped the needle cap on the floor and started searching for it. He gave up the search and inserted a needle in my left arm and attached a bag of saline. They didn't seem to have a sense of urgency – at least not like I remembered in the medical shows I grew up watching as a kid.

"Don't we have to get to the hospital?" I pleaded.

"We'll get there soon."

"Can we get going now?"

I was scared. Terrified, really. It was late, they appeared tired – I realize now they were doing a great job. But at one in the morning, wondering if I was going to die in my driveway, I didn't see it. Finally, one suggested to the other that maybe they should get going. He jumped into the front and started the engine.

I have seen many ambulances racing through town, and always have given them a wide berth. This ride let me know how important that was. They "hauled ass" to the hospital. Judy said she tried to follow us but they outran her in spades. That EMT dude could drive.

Through the entire drive I kept thinking: *If I can get to the hospital, I'll be all right. If I just hold on'till then. Please God, let me hold on.* That Catholic training was subconscious, automatic. I didn't realize until later just how deep they were.

The ambulance pulled in front of the hospital, backed up, and when the rear doors opened, emergency room personnel in blue scrubs greeted me. One of the men gave them my vitals while they pulled me out of the ambulance, lowered the legs of the gurney and rolled me through the automatic doors into the hospital.

"Take him to ER 3," I heard someone say.

"Do you understand what I am saying?" a nurse asked me.

"Yes," I replied. I was thinking normally, but everything was a bit hazy.

Once in the room, an ER doctor rushed in. A blur of back-and-forth conversations between the medical personnel grew from a slight chatter to a cacophony of background noises while I lay there, spinning, and the increasing volume of my wretched headache. They took my vitals again and finally the doctor's voice cut through the noise to say, "Inject Demerol into the IV." Within ten seconds I started to feel less anxious. Then a wave of calm swept came over and through me. I didn't care about the noise. Maybe I was going to live. Maybe I had gotten to the hospital in time. Maybe.

*I started to feel less anxious. Then a wave of calm came over me.*

I didn't care anymore. My headache was gone. I was still spinning, but it didn't bother me. The doctor kept asking me questions, but they became echoes in a long tunnel ... something in the background of my Demerol high. I threw up. They gave me something for the nausea.

I heard the doctor say she thought it was a stroke, but that my case was unusual. I was conscious, lucid. They had a treatment for stroke patients, the drug tPP, but she was hesitant to give it to me. She thought that maybe they should get an MRI before proceeding any further.

I'll always be grateful for her caution and insight. I later learned that if I had taken the treatment it could have worsened my condition and possibly been catastrophic for me.

More echoes in the background. I heard Judy arrive and they let her and Daisy (our Malti-Poo service dog) sit in the room with me. I looked over at her, smiled.

I thought then that I would live. I was not going to die, yet. Hope started to peek above the horizon. And then everything was a blur. I would live, and that was all that mattered.

I closed my eyes. It all felt like a dream.

Judy told me she called our good friends Bob and Cherie. They rushed to the hospital at six in the morning and brought coffee for her. She and Daisy had been sitting in the ER room and then the hospital room all night long.

The next clear thought was my being in a hospital room, beeping and mechanical sounds in the background. Alone. What had happened? Why was I there? My head was still spinning, but less. I tried to sit up. Couldn't.

The left side of my body was … weak, I guessed. *I'll try a little later.* Right then, I wanted to go back to sleep. I did.

The nurse came in, woke me up and shot me with a tranquilizer. They needed an MRI. This was for me to get through it. I think the MRI was the equivalent of being in a coffin for thirty minutes. I say think, because I have almost no memory of the experience. I didn't care.

Judy walked into the room. I felt her there before I saw her. Opening my eyes, I could see the lines of concern etched on her face, although there seemed to be an attempt to "put on the happy face." It didn't work. She half-smiled, sat down.

"Hi, honey," I said, words sounding a bit slurred to me.

"Hi there."

"What happened?"

"Doctors said you had a stroke, although they don't know what kind, exactly."

I looked out the window; it looked like mid-morning. Blue sky. Cotton white clouds. I started to remember the previous night.

*I had a stroke?*

"How do you feel?" she asked.

I guess that is the first question everyone thinks to ask a patient in the hospital. Almost reactive. Still, it seemed like a reasonable question to me.

"I don't know."

I tried to raise my left arm; it was weak, but I could rub my nose. My left leg would only lift a few inches above the bed.

"I had a stroke?"

Judy nodded. I thought for a moment. Taking inventory of my body and mind, I was thinking, *that's good*. In the hospital bed, I tried to sit up, but could not. My head could turn. I could feel cold, which it clearly was in that hospital room.

An unwelcome thought came to me like an unkept stranger asking for money. Unable to be ignored. I remembered the hushed tones used for others when talking about strokes. Then I understood. My life from that moment forward was going to be different. How? I was unsure. But I knew it. Could feel it. Because I was still drugged up from the previous evening, the clarity of my thinking was dulled, yet I sensed that there was a long road ahead that would test everything I had believed in.

From the first book my father gave me, "The Magic of Believing" by Claude Bristol, to Dale Carnegie and dozens of other self-help gurus, I had come to believe that I was at my core a positive person; that the will to overcome, and my own thoughts controlled my reality. But it is easy to be positive when all is well. Not so easy when the chips are down. My chips were all in. I did not have a choice. The road before me would be a test. I either believed I could get better, and make the process a positive and uplifting one, or not.

*I either believed I would get better, and make the process a positive and uplifting one, or not.*

Judy also shared how my friend Jon from Florida drove to the house and was helping her out there. That took a load of worry off my shoulders.

The nurse came and went with a handful of pills. I took them. Some of them must have been for pain. My headache, still throbbing, subsided. I felt dreamy.

"What did the doctors say about it?" I asked Judy.

"No word yet. I went home when they knocked you out for the MRI, cleaned up and came right back. They said a doctor would see you this morning."

*Good,* I whispered to myself. I had a lot of questions. The most pressing was, *How bad is it?* I like to get the worst-case scenario and then go from there. That has always helped me in business, and although I was not sure why, I felt knowing the worst that *could* happen would make me feel better. At least I would know.

I smiled at Judy. "I'm glad you're here."

Later that day, a doctor came in and introduced herself as a neurologist at the hospital. She had charts and a pad under her right arm. Judy was there with Daisy (her cute little Malti-Poo).

"Mr. Woods," she started, "I've looked at your charts and your MRI. It appears that your left rear artery, called the vertebral, is completely blocked. What happened was once this closed off, the blood flow to your brain was reduced. There is a blood vessel called The Circle of Willis that all four of the arteries to your brain feed into. It is a sort of an equalizer to make sure blood is distributed evenly to your brain.

"Because of the blockage, the few seconds that it took for the blood to be evenly distributed cut off some blood to the nerve center located in your spinal column. This is what caused your stroke. It is very unusual to have this kind of stroke. Usually, it is the carotid arteries that become blocked. In any event, it appears from the MRI to be a 100% blockage."

She looked through the charts. Because of all the medications, especially the Percocet, I was straining to understand. Even though I was lying in the bed, my mind leaned toward her.

"What is perplexing is that your blood pressure is normal, your cholesterol is fine, and quite frankly, we don't know why this happened. You seem to be in perfect health. We'll run some more tests, but at this point we just don't know."

"Is there anything I can do?" I asked. I immediately realized that may have sounded humorous given my current condition.

She furrowed her brow. "Well, in normal cases we would have a slew of drugs for you to take. In this case, we have you on a few of them, but at this point the main thing is to take a baby aspirin once you get home. We have your blood pressure high right now, which is part of the recovery treatment. But in a few days, we'll lower it and hopefully you'll be able to start getting some physical therapy. How are your headaches?"

"Better, since I just took something. But my head is spinning, and I am seeing double."

"We'll keep you out of pain, and hopefully give you something to help the vertigo. In the meantime, get some rest. You have been through a lot."

She stood, tapped the side railing of my bed and left.

I watched her walk out the door, a pause that lasted a few heartbeats.

Judy looked at me. "That seemed pretty positive."

"It did. Now I just have to get better." I didn't realize how long a road that would be. But something within me was determined to get through it. No matter what it took.

"Honey, I told some of our friends and they want to come see you."

"Perhaps a bit later," I replied.

"Okay. They just want you to know they are concerned."

"I get that. Tell them thank you."

"Do you need anything?"

"Yeah. To get back to where I was before last night." I laughed. My sense of humor was still intact. Even if my body wasn't.

"You will," she replied. And I knew she was right. I would.

The next few days were a whirlwind of friends visiting, doctors checking in, medications being swallowed, and tests. I loved having my friends visit. It is quite monotonous to be lying in bed, unable to really move to get comfortable, with only the TV to keep you company. Company. I found TV to be a placebo to stop the mind from having any meaningful thoughts—electronic heroin for the numbing of the mind. I watched for a couple of hours and turned it off. Permanently.

> TV really is a placebo for the mind… it was electronic heroin…

It seemed friends came at all hours the entire three days I was in the hospital. And it was welcome.

"Yes, I had a stroke."

"No, I don't know when I will be getting back home."

"Yes, the food here is good."

"No, the doctors still do not know why it happened."

"Yes, please keep me in your prayers."

I love every one of them. Their intentions were pure, and the face time made my life bearable throughout my tenure in the small, private room. It's hard to explain, but the fact that I had friends that loved me gave me an inner strength, a primal urge, to get better. That coupled with Judy's love and concern were paramount to my remaining positive and hopeful.

On day two, a neurosurgeon came in and introduced himself. He began friendly but matter of fact.

"I've looked at your MRIs and all your charts. You have a 100% blockage in your left rear artery, the vertebral. If it was 90%, we could do something about that. But since it is 100%, there is nothing we can do surgically. The problem is if we do go in and loosen something, then it will cause more damage than you already have suffered, and in fact could kill you. I wanted to come by and tell you."

I was dealing with a number of symptoms...

Then he reached down, grabbed my arm and smiled. "Good luck." He turned and left the room.

*Good luck?*

*What the heck does that mean? So, there is no way to fix what is wrong with me?* At that point I was dealing with a number of symptoms: double vision, vertigo, inability to walk straight, almost complete loss of strength in my left leg, and the inability to urinate (they inserted a catheter—most painful).

And, because of all the opioids, I was constipated. He was telling me I was on my own as far as healing was concerned.

*Thanks for nothing.*

I used the power-bed to lay my head back, so I could see the ceiling and think. *What am I going to do? What are my options? I don't know anything about strokes.*

Except... I did.

I remembered writing a story years ago with my friend Sheila about a doctor named Jacob who worked in the University of Oregon. He was dealing with stroke patients. His theory involved using DMSO (Dimethyl Sulfoxide) to clear the blood vessels, and he was very successful. Maybe that could work? I knew I couldn't try it until I was released; and I also knew from the multitude of "sales people" for the physical therapy rehab locations who visited me that I had five or six weeks of physical therapy ahead before I would be going home. That seemed like a long time.

> *I had five or six weeks of physical therapy ahead of me before I would be going home.*

Four days after entering the emergency room at the hospital, I was released to go to rehab at Springhill Rehabilitation Center in Mobile. I was transferred to an ambulance and taken there. During the trip, my blood pressure rose to 180 over 140. They told the admitting nurse about it. She said they were so busy that my blood pressure would have to be over 200 before they could spare someone to see me. I was pretty sure that was not indicative of good patient care and wondered if the rehab program I was about to enter was any better.

I found out soon enough.

"You will have to do physical therapy for two hours per day while you are here," the nurse said. "We'll split it into two one-hour periods, if you like."

I liked that. The room at Springhill was small and utilitarian. They did not go over budget with the bed or decorations. The PT times were 10 until 11, and then 2 until 3. The rest of the time was simply laying in bed. I was severely cross-eyed from the stroke, so could not read, one of my passionate obsessions. So, I was resigned to simply think. I say *"simply"* in jest, since it is very difficult to think about what you want, instead of letting your mind take you where it wants to go. I battled negative thoughts twenty-two hours every day.

*Am I really going to get better?*

*How long will this take?*

*What if I don't get better?*

*Wait! Do not entertain those kinds of thoughts.*

*What if my d**k doesn't work again?* This last one is a guy thing, I know. But I had a catheter in it and half my body was out of commission. It was a relevant thought. After all, I was only sixty-five years old, with years of (hopefully) great sex lying ahead of me. At least, I hoped so.

PT was very rudimentary: pedal a sit-down bike, fold clothes, try to walk with a walker. I was still in a wheelchair, and these stand-up walking exercises really challenged me. I was leaning to the left, almost in vertigo, and the step after step—even the few feet requested of me—was difficult. Excruciatingly so. Added to this was an eyepatch they gave me to help with the double vision and vertigo. No depth perception.

For a majority of the time, the PT therapists were all looking at their phones, once they gave me (and everyone else) a task to accomplish. I could have rolled out of the room in my wheelchair flapping my arms like a duck and they would probably not have noticed. There was no observation, unless I made a loud noise or interrupted their viewing of the phone to inform them I had finished the task. It was like this the entire month I was there.

My load of medications continued. I was still taking 40 mcg of Percocet a day, along with five other medications prescribed to help me with a few problems I was experiencing, the most annoying of which were non-stop hiccups. These included blood thinners, tranquilizers, cholesterol medications, prostrate reducers and a baby aspirin. After a few weeks, I got them (the hiccups) under control. The Percocet helped the headaches tremendously, and also helped me sleep.

*I was still taking 40 mcg of Percocet a day... blood thinners, tranquilizers, cholesterol medications, prostrate reducers and a baby aspirin*

Our friends pitched in and divided up among themselves the task of getting Judy to and from Springfield (about an hour away from Fairhope) on a daily basis. Our friend Tamlin organized this system, and it seemed every day Judy and another friend would come visit me, which helped with the doldrums I was fighting. Those visits were welcomed and cherished.

My leg started getting a bit stronger, and by the time I left I was able to use a walker, although it was tenuous. We ordered a wheelchair for the house. The walker came from Emmy's, a thrift shop in Fairhope, that has a free loaner program for Fairhope residents. I was not surprised as this is the nature of the towns' spirit where we live.

One surprising aspect of this stroke: On the last day of my physical therapy, I was allowed to go into the bathroom and shave. In my wheelchair, I turned on the hot water, reached my right hand under the stream and it felt cold. Strange, I thought. I waited a minute more, put my finger into it and the same – it was cold. I used my left hand and almost burned myself. The right side of my body feels hot as cold. Is that not interesting? When I shared this experience with the neurologist, he found it fascinating as well—he had actually never heard of it before.

It was surreal coming home almost five weeks from the time the stroke happened. Memories were vivid of my having been wheeled out on the gurney, and here I was walking in (with the walker). I was ecstatic. I was home. I felt a grounding. Judy had the house cleaned, and it felt new, welcoming. Friends had brought my computer from the upstairs office down to the ground floor for me, so I could work, which, in the past month, had fallen into arrears.

Home.

I remember looking in the bathroom mirror and seeing my 'pirate' eye patch over my left eye. I looked, well, 'piratee'. I laughed. Eight years earlier I had written a sequel to Robert Louis Stevenson's Treasure Island. And here I was sporting an eye patch with a skull and cross bones embroidered across it.

It is hard to imagine being in a hospital and wondering if you would ever get back home – if you have not been in such a situation. I had wondered a lot of things: *Would I walk again? Would I be able to see again* (I still had terrible double vision)?*Would I be able to write again?* I wanted to be in my own bed, under my own blankets with my head nestled in my own pillow, which I promptly did.

Unlike my snap decision to not watch TV in the rehab center, I decided to stop taking all of my medications. I had planned this for weeks. They would not let me stop taking them in rehab, so this was the first opportunity to quit. I took the five bottles, placed them into a cabinet and told myself that was it.

Part of the reason was my bladder. I felt the Percocet and Flowmax were keeping me from having normal bladder release, and they instructed me on how to self-catheterize (yes, it is as awful as it sounds) whenever I had to empty my bladder. Worse, I needed Judy to help me.

*It took three days, but I was finally able to urinate on my own*

I also decided to crawl up the stairs to my office instead of using the new office downstairs. I dragged my walker up with me. I was determined not to give in to my 'temporary' limitations.

It took three days, but I was finally able to urinate on my own, and I considered that a great success. In fact, I took it as a sign that eventually all could be well.

Two things happened during those first few days that also contributed to that positive thought: my friend Freddie coming over and a home physical therapist named Brian who showed up to help me. Freddie was unique. He told me about his recovery from a tragic fall in his garage.

"John," he said, "here is what you have to do. If you are told to walk for a half hour a day, you walk an hour. If they say do ten reps of your leg exercise, do twenty. In other words, you need to push yourself as far and hard as you can. In this way, you will get better quicker and sooner."

"Makes sense," I said.

"And do not give up," Freddie added. "You can beat this. I did."

Brian, the physical therapist, came to the house. I was expecting a big, muscular fellow with no sense of humor. He was thin and looked very average. His calm, pleasant uplifting demeanor gave me hope.

With an assuring voice, he said: "We're going to go slowly and build up your balance and ability to get around the house at first," Brian said. "You have to trust me on this. Things will get better. I am not able to tell you when or how long this will take, but it will get better if you practice what I show you and work consistently at it."

During this time, I still had two additional problems to figure out. They stemmed from the neurologist at the hospital telling me he "hopes it works out." That was not good enough for me.

The first problem was my sight.

A friend who was also an acupuncturist (and a stroke survivor) came to the house and told me the following:

"John, I believe that acupuncture can help with your balance and your eyesight. It did with me. The secret is treating the nerves around your eyes – stimulating them – to correct the abnormality."

*I had a great deal of secondhand knowledge of acupuncture, but had never tried it*

I had a great deal of secondhand knowledge of acupuncture, having read about it, but had never tried it before. I was ready to try it. A few weeks later I met him at his office, and we had the first treatment. He told me I would not feel the needles (I did, but they were not overly painful), and inserted about twenty-five or so on my weak left leg and around my eyes. It is a bit unnerving seeing needles peripherally around your eyes, but I was committed to trying anything. I went to see Dr. Stump twice a week.

The second problem was oxygen. My brain was simply not getting enough.

Part of the advantage of lying around the hospital twenty-two hours a day with nothing to do is getting in touch with your thoughts and memories. One such memory was an article I had read about returning Middle East vets who had traumatic brain injuries from explosions they had experienced. A VA (I forgot where) was trying hyperbaric oxygen chambers to try to re-oxygenate the brain of these injured vets and repair it. They had some observable and intermittent successes.

I reasoned that a stroke was similar in the sense that a lack of oxygen to the brain caused the same type of injury. But what do you do to find (and pay for) a hyperbaric chamber??

I called around and found that unless I had a "covered" injury (such as diabetes or open wounds), I could not use the chambers in medical centers or hospitals. Not even paying cash. They only allowed insurance reimbursable treatments such as open wounds from diabetes. I found a private provider in the city of Daphne who had a wonderful chamber that I could sit up in. Only one problem– it cost two-hundred dollars per hour.

Further research led me to Dr. Harch in Louisiana, who was doing extensive work on strokes and hyperbaric chambers. I contacted him. The program was for forty hours in the chamber over a period of months, at a cost of over two-hundred dollars per hour; plus living expenses, since I would have to temporarily live near the chamber in order to participate. His program was intended to prove through peer-reviewed studies that the chambers had more than a palliative effect on stroke recovery.

Undeterred, I remained hopeful.

I finally found a chiropractor in Gulf Shores who was using hyperbaric oxygen therapy and would rent me the chamber for sixty dollars an hour, if I purchased ten hours at a time. Happy to pay, Judy and I made a two-hour drive to get there and return three days a week.

The chiropractor, Dr. Sabal, shared a number of stories that stroke survivors like myself had experienced.

*I felt that this would help with my sight and balance*

"After a few weeks they started walking better" she said. Then after a month or so they started driving again. Vision improved. It is not a cut-and-dry formula – each patient is different. But at least you will have the hope that you can get better."

There it was again. Hope. It was all I had to go on. Yet somewhere deep inside myself, perhaps my intuition, I felt that this would help with my sight and balance. I had already seen an ophthalmologist who tested me extensively and told me there was nothing they could do about my double vision. My eyes were too far out of alignment. I needed hope.

The chamber is made of a special polymer tube that you zip yourself within. When I first saw it, I was hesitant. I wasn't claustrophobic (at least, I didn't think I was), but I didn't really know. The chamber was about three feet around and eight feet long. You zip up (actually the chiropractor zips you in) and then you hear an air pump start to pressurize air.

The principle is pretty simple. These chambers were designed to oxygenate the body of divers who had the bends from coming to the surface too quickly. My problem was not getting enough oxygen to my brain and to repair the damage already caused by a lack of oxygen because of the vertebral artery being blocked. The chambers pressurized up to eighty feet below the surface of the ocean and pushed the oxygen directly into your skin and capillaries and could get oxygen directly to your brain.

*Being within the tube is not scary at all*

So the theory goes. I was willing to test the theory.

Being within the tube is not scary at all. In fact, perhaps it is primordial in the sense you feel protected, almost as if you were in a cocoon, safe from the world and its troubles. I found that I would think, not worry, when I was inside. And sleep, too.

The hours passed rather quickly, and I started looking forward to my hour in the chamber, although the drives were not so much fun. Judy was the driver, since I could not see clearly unless I closed one eye, which was terrible for depth perception.

One of the first things I did upon returning home was contact Dr. Jacob at Oregon State University. I had written an article over twenty years earlier about his research into DMSO and strokes. A friend had suffered a massive stroke and was considered beyond help. My friend Sheila and I put him in touch with Dr. Jacob and he went through the treatment, which included daily injections of DMSO. He recovered completely.

Contacting Oregon State University, I learned Dr. Jacob had died, and his son referred me to an ND (Naturopathic Doctor) who had taken over his practice and lived in Washington State. I called and spoke with him. I explained what had happened, that I had a 100% blockage of my vertebral artery, and no hope of clearing it out. At least not yet.

"I think you should rub DMSO over the area of the artery to start the release of the blockage," he said.

"Okay," I replied. "But the problem is that if anything releases inside the artery, it will go directly into my brain. That is why they will not operate on me – there is no way to assure that nothing will release from the artery during the operation."

"Oh, I see." There was a long silence. "Maybe then you should take CoQ10 and a few other things to see if they will help."

*See if they will help? What does that mean?* I don't mind being a guinea pig if the treatment makes sense (I was going through acupuncture and hyperbaric oxygen treatments already), but unless you can state a valid reason for a treatment working, I was not about to do it. I knew that with a cerebral hemorrhagic stroke the DMSO was truly a miracle, yet in my case it would probably do the exact opposite. I reached a dead end as far as DMSO was concerned.

A dead end. But in my search, I was relieved to find that the stroke did not affect my logic, reasoning or ability to carry on with the daily activity of living.

During this time, I closed escrow on our home (using my walker to arrive at the escrow office to sign all the documents), started remodeling the deck for a porch, built a pier wharf and boathouse, edited and published books, and bought a new car to make the drives to and from Gulf Shores.

*Within another month, I was able to start driving.*

I went to acupuncture twice a week, physical therapy twice a week, and oxygen therapy three times a week.

I was creating hope.

About two months later I first started noticing my eyes were getting better. Subtle at first, but noticeably better. I could watch TV without closing my left eye. Progress. Hope.

Within another month, I was able to start driving. It was difficult, but I could do it. Judy was relieved. She could ride with me now to Gulf Shores instead of driving.

Progress.

In January, I was speaking with my cousin Brian called with terrible news: my cousin, his sister Linda, had died of cancer. In the course of the conversation, I mentioned my progress and how the hyperbaric chamber was really helping me. He asked if I could buy one.

"Yes, Brian. In fact, I checked them out at first before going to the chiropractor. The number-one manufacturer is actually within fifty miles of you in Santa Fe Springs (California)."

"How much are they?" he asked.

"About ten thousand dollars," I replied.

There was a pause on the phone for a few seconds.

"How about if I go and look at them for you?" he said.

*"Hey John, I bought you one. It will ship out in a few days."*

*Great. I could probably afford one*, I thought, *but it would be tight*.

The next day Brian called:

"Hey, John, I bought you one. It will ship out in a few days."

I was dumbfounded. "Really?"

"Yeah. I'm going to get one, too."

Tears formed in my eyes and my voice cracked. "Brian, thank you so much."

"No problem, Cuz. Just keep getting better."

The chamber arrived a week later, and from then on, I was in it every day. I spoke with a nurse at the factory who suggested that I mega-dose–get in twice a day, at least for the first month. I followed her direction and it made a world of difference. The double vision completely disappeared. My balance was better, and energy level almost back to normal.

I was convinced that, unlike that exercise machine people commit to and a month later becomes a coat hanger, this chamber would be used by me, perhaps the rest of my life.

I continued the acupuncture and PT for about nine months. It has been four months since I stopped both, with little appreciable change in the energy or cognitive functions.

I feel pretty well.

One day I went to see my neurologist who had been checking in and seeing me since I had arrived at rehab in Spanish Fort. When he walked in the exam room, he seemed shocked—I assumed in a good way. He asked what I had been doing, and I explained the treatments I had done, with special emphasis on the oxygen chamber.

Incredulous, he said. "Well, you've made a believer out of me. I never would have thought that a hyperbaric chamber could make such a difference. You look great."

*"...you've made a believer out of me. I never would have thought that a hyperbaric chamber could make such a difference. You look great."*

What he didn't say was that the outcome for a stroke with one artery 100% blocked was not good. Simple fluid dynamics. 75% blood and oxygen flow versus 100%. The only thing he could recommend was to increase my blood pressure to try to compensate; but we both agreed that too much blood pressure is what could cause another stroke. He admitted there was no literature that said it would work anyway.

Today, if you walked behind me, you would notice I still "list" slightly to the left. As to my general health, I am healthy and almost completely back to my old self. Not quite as energetic yet, but getting better every week. I still feel hot as cold on my left side, and I have no pain sensation on that side either. Easily lived with. Easily compensated.

Living in the South, my takeaway from the whole "spell" (a Southern term for stroke and other maladies) is this: You sometimes have to go outside the box to get better. Medicine is fantastic for emergencies and other life-threatening events, but not the cure-all for an event like a stroke.

> *I had no choice. I had to take charge of my health.*

I had no choice. I had to take charge of my health. The neurosurgeon had wished me good luck. But I wanted more than luck. My prognosis early on was not good, and my health and cognitive abilities would have rapidly dwindled to a point I do not even want to think about.

The bigger lesson is this: if being lucky is defined as following my thoughts and intuition to find a solution to my problem, then I was lucky. But I also think that by pioneering my own solutions I discovered treatments that can help others in similar situations.

Furthermore, my responsibility and commitment is to share my story. When somebody tells me they, or a loved one, has had a stroke, I suggest they find a hyperbaric oxygen chamber (or use mine if close by), get DMSO (if it is a hemorrhagic stroke) and follow Dr. Jacob's procedure (easily found on the Internet). I recommend they find a qualified acupuncturist and get competent physical therapy.

And most importantly, to get their thoughts under control.

As I mentioned earlier, it is easy to be positive when all is well, less so when the chips are down. I believe that keeping my thoughts focused on getting better was a tremendous help in my journey. I mentioned earlier Dale Carnegie, but the real help for me was a course called *The Master Key Course*. I provide a link in the resources section.

Finally, I suspect most of us. whenever we find our life is in danger, call on God for help. My Catholicism and faith, especially instilled by Mother, gave me a belief in something bigger than me. And hope, although I was never a devout Catholic since my teenage years. Now that I am out of danger and able to reflect, I credit my Father for introducing me to the concept that thoughts and intentions play a critical role in the healing process. I still battle with it every day, although they are small skirmishes and getting much easier.

Beyond all the opportunities that modern medicine promises, behind all the advancements announced every day, the decision on what to do is still yours. You MUST take charge of your own health. Your destiny is in YOUR hands.

All of these methods can lead to a level of recovery that allows for a joyous, wonderful life even after what seemed to be a tragedy.

I know.

I have been through it.

**Resources**

*Hyperbaric Chambers:*

https://www.oxyhealth.com/

There are others, some less expensive. BUT, this is the best. I looked on youtube and found that you can build one for less than a couple of hundred dollars. Check that out too.

*Acupuncturists:*

https://aaaomonline.org/

*Physical Therapists:*

http://www.apta.org/

*Supplements:*

Magnesium, Calcium and Potassium 2-AEP

Hans Nieper MD Formula –

Available at Amazon

*Pre and Pro Biotics:*

http://microbiomeplus.com/

*Enzymes:*

Essential enzymes 500mg

Available at Amazon

*CBD oil:*

This is a problem, because I am using 1-part THC to 1-part CBD, which is illegal in half the country. I do know you need to get it from the cannabis plant, not the hemp plant.

*Reading:*

'A stroke of Midnight' by John L. Stump

"The Magic of Believing" by Claude Bristle

"How to Win Friends and Influence People" by Dale Carnegie

"Think and Grow Rich' by Napoleon Hill

*Course:*

The Master Key Course

www.TheMasterKeyCourse.com

**Further research**

Dr. Paul G. Harch:

http://www.hbot.com/about-practice

Dr. Stanley W. Jacob:

https://www.jacoblab.com/

## Epilogue

My stroke was unusual. In fact, my neurologist had never seen one like mine before, neither had a friend of mine who had been a nurse for forty-years. Having said that, the protocols I have suggested will still help everyone who has a stroke.

HOWEVER, if it is a hemorrhagic stroke, there are additional things you need to consider, including blood thinners and statins until you get your body under control. I suggest you go to:

https://www.stroke.org/

Learn what they recommend.

Additional suggestions.

- Get your mercury amalgam fillings replaced.
- Change your diet (not to vegetarian)
- Exercise. (Try walking)
- Get your body weight under control. Easiest way is to eat half of what you normally do and see if that helps. Add pre and pro biotics and enzymes.
- Make sure your home and work environments are not toxic – especially with mold.
- When you get your teeth cleaned or hair washed at a salon, use an airline pillow for supporting your neck.

And lastly, treat your physician like an auto mechanic. In other words, question what they say and use your intuition along with facts to decide your future treatment options. If they are wrong, it is YOU that will pay for it.

**Hyperbaric Oxygen Chamber**

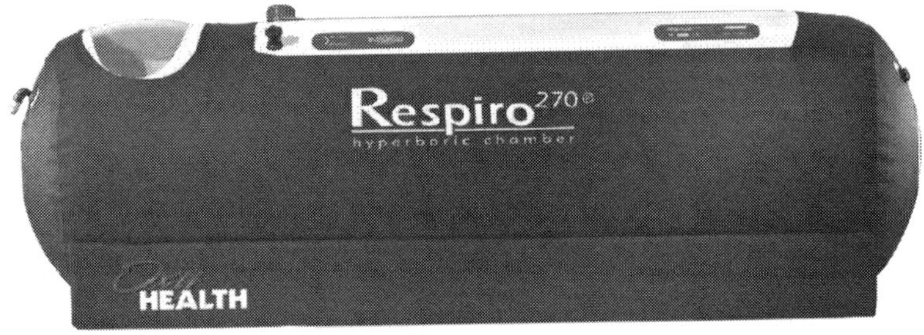


You can get out of this by yourself, but I haven't figured out a way to get into it and zip it up by myself.

Is it claustrophobic?

Not for me.

It has a window on top and at both ends. And if I were feeling uncomfortable, I can turn off the pump and be out, by myself, in two minutes.

And, it certainly beats the alternative outcome I was facing.

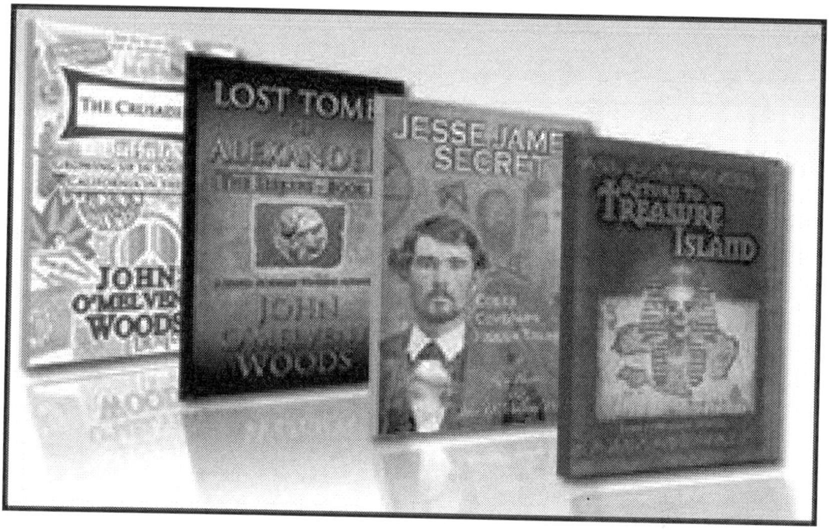
TREASURE
ISLAND



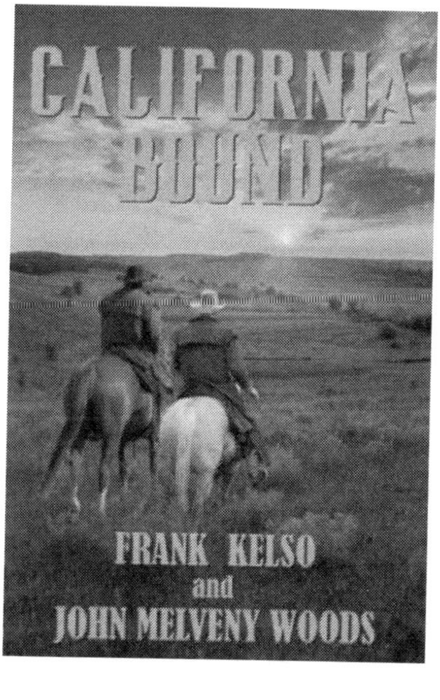
CALIFORNIA
BOUND
FRANK KELSO
and
JOHN MELVENY WOODS

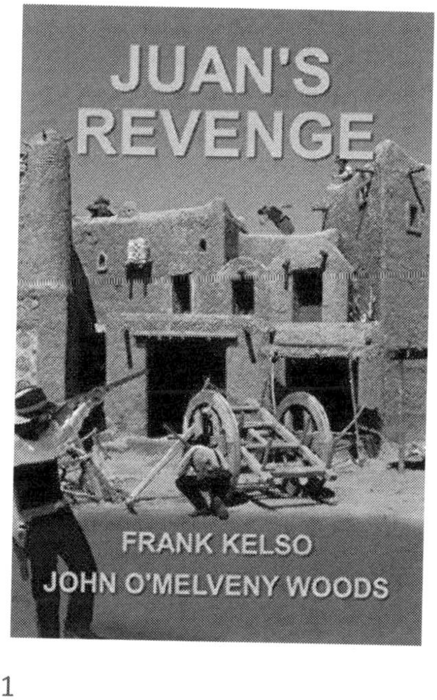
JUAN'S
REVENGE
FRANK KELSO
JOHN O'MELVENY WOODS

Made in the USA
Monee, IL
06 November 2026

68143264R00025